MAINTAIN YOUR HEALTH IN
COLLEGE YEARS

Find Out How?

Nam Nguyen

authorHOUSE®

AuthorHouse™ UK
1663 Liberty Drive
Bloomington, IN 47403 USA
www.authorhouse.co.uk
Phone: 0800.197.4150

Published by AuthorHouse 10/06/2016

ISBN: 978-1-5246-6401-5 (sc)
ISBN: 978-1-5246-6403-9 (hc)
ISBN: 978-1-5246-6402-2 (e)

Print information available on the last page.

Any people depicted in stock imagery provided by Thinkstock are models,
and such images are being used for illustrative purposes only.
Certain stock imagery © Thinkstock.

This book is printed on acid-free paper.

CONTENTS

PREFACE

The teenage is the most beautiful time of human life as it is accompanied with friends, new adventures, excitements, achievements, and dreams.

All of us have our own dreams and goals at this age and together with them, come the hurdles and our own battles. Now, most of you might think that I referred as 'hurdles' and 'battles' to the exams, tournaments, and competitions. No, the real hurdle of our life is to stay healthy at all times. This does not differ in teenage as well. To reach your goals, to party with friends, to do sports and even to pass exams with flying colors, you need to be in good health.

This book is a guide for all college students, teenagers and even for parents to learn the importance of health in youth. It will reveal many secrets and also will give you many tips. Many young adults ignore the complete definition of health; they either focus on their physical health or may be only on social health. But, this book will redefine the whole image you have about maintaining your good health.

Starting from physical health to the sexual health of teenagers are reviewed, discussed and given advices on. Not only about the health but also this book speaks about stress, depression, alcoholism, smoking and many other problems the youth face in this modern world. Some health issues are still remained silent and never spoken about. Lack of knowledge may make them worse. That is why this book can be a basic guide to teach your young adult about sexual health as well.

This book is written in order to help the readers get enough knowledge and to help them to lead a healthy lifestyle. The information in this book is put together after doing a thorough research on scientific findings, medical and health literature and medical advices from professionals. I would rather call this as an access point to free health advice as well. You will find answers to your questions in each chapter and that is why THIS BOOK MUST BE A BOOK THAT YOU HAVE AT HOME.

I hope you will enjoy reading, studying, finding answers and also sharing this book with your friends, family, and acquaintances. Acquiring a good knowledge about health and spreading it, is one of the best things you could do to make the future generations healthy, strong and happy!

IMPORTANCE OF PHYSICAL HEALTH AT THIS AGE

According to World Health Organization (WHO) health is defined as 'a state of complete physical, mental, and social well-being and not merely the absence of disease or infirmity' and the physical health has always been the most widely spoken component when it comes to health.

The physical well-being of a person is important at every age. But, when considering the physical activeness and related lifestyle, it is well known that physical activeness is really high in the youth. Compared to the adult age and elderly age, the people in youth keep on moving, partying, traveling, enrolling in sports as well as participating in many other activities. Therefore, a proper physical health and fitness are necessary to live and enjoy the youth to the fullest.

An optimum physical health is built up by many other co-factors such as healthy weight maintenance, physical fitness, proper nutrition, optimum growth, disease prevention and so on. Therefore, it is not only the weight and fitness a college student should be worried about but, also about all the other things that are necessary to maintain a physical well-being.

Think about all those college students you know, how busy, exciting, fun and full of spirit their lives are. But, if one of them keeps on catching colds frequently or become overweight or too slim to even enroll in sports and other activities, how that might affect his life and goals? Think if they do not have a proper nutrition and needs alcohol for every special reason, their lives wouldn't be any more exciting and indifferent. Yes, all these things matter when it comes to the best time of your life – The Youth – The age of discovering the world, discovering yourself, achieving the goals, falling in love and being an inspiration for the next generation.

If we ask many adults, they would miss being a college student. They will cherish those moments when they enjoyed time with friends doing crazy things, when they ate whatever they liked, when they were the stars of the college football team or cheerleading team or how they were smart, achieving the highest grades in exams. Yes, life is the most exciting at this time period. But, you should not remember the much it is exciting, it is that much challenging as well.

One of the main challenges a college student faces, other than exams, getting selected to school sports teams and getting into a university, is maintaining the physical wellbeing. In spite of being among hundreds of students in the college for more than six hours (who might have infections), eating whatever they get when they are out, functioning the brain almost continuously for 12-16 hours and sleepless nights cramming for exams, a college students must be healthy enough to get up the next day and go out with the aim of achieving their goals. Isn't it the biggest challenge a person would ever have? Yes, it is. The only thing is that we haven't given a thought about it yet!

Don't worry! This book will guide you on how to be in proper physical health, how to overcome the physical challenges and how you can face the life with more optimism. We have got answers for all of your questions. As this little knowledge packed in this book will guide you and your friends to live the college life to the maximum, I am quite sure, you will very soon witness the blessing of being a healthy youth.

IMPORTANCE OF MENTAL HEALTH AT THIS AGE

The brain functions the maximum at this age and millions of neurons work every single second changing their chemistry to form new memories and to transfer already created memories from short term memory to long term memory. Actually, all parts of the brain including communication centers of the brain functions in a very high level at this age.

The listening, speech, writing, creativity and also the logical mind is always active and functions in its maximum capacity. What a huge workload is that for a single brain? A single nerve transmission makes hundreds of chemical reactions and involves thousands of nerves, which need enough of energy and an optimal healthy biochemical atmosphere so that there won't be any disturbances.

Brain is a part of human body, which is very complex, but, it is also the most important organ as it controls the complete body; the hormones, activities and even the entire metabolism. The brain keeps on forming new neuronal connections every second and this is how the brain works. Our five sensory organs keep on gathering information and our brain process them by eliminating the less important information. The main information is then stored in the brain. Each information, which is received from each sensory organ, makes a new memory so that the same memory will be formed in many pathways with many links. Once you need to recall this information, all these pathways will help you in recalling what you need. As there are many links formed, there cannot be any information loss within the brain.

Isn't our brain super extraordinary? Yes, it is. The human brain and its functions cannot be completely understood. It is, of course, interesting and fun to know how your brain works. But, what is more important than that is, getting to know how to keep your brain functions and the mental health at its optimum level.

Especially in the youth, when the brain functions the most, it is our responsibility to take care of our brain. A proper nutrition, a good night sleep, brain exercises and enough of brain relaxation is necessary to have a healthy mind.

The new discoveries, the vast amount of knowledge, the problems and the stress at this age should be perceived and managed in a healthy way. For this, it is important that college students have enough knowledge on how to maintain their mental health. This is the best time to introduce relaxation techniques such as yoga, meditation, aromatherapy and reflexology into your lifestyle.

Being a member in youth communities and being a part of the clubs which focus on increasing memory power and even counseling with your college counselor, when you feel you need someone to talk to, shouldn't be underestimated as things that aren't necessary for your life. A smart student always seeks help when he/she is confused and it is never an act of weakness but is an act of smartness.

IMPORTANCE OF SOCIAL WELL-BEING

The college life is all about making new friends, meeting new people and connecting with people around the world. At this age, it is essential that you make a healthy relationship with your parents, family, friends, teachers and others around you. Even though some think that connecting with people is an art, actually it is a part of health and well-being.

Social well being surely is a component of health, but, it fully depends on physical and mental well-being. As you know a good physique and a good appearance attract people. But it is not only that which matters. A good personality, intelligence, creativity, and humor are also important to make very good connections with people around you. All these things are characteristics of a healthy young adult.

A college is a place where the students enroll in many extracurricular activities such as different competitions within the college and inter-college activities, which will require you to build a good social life. Hence, social well-being is important as much as the physical and mental well-being. Some mental disorders such as anxiety, depression and mood disorders can stay undetected and yet might affect the social life of a person in a great manner. Mental health is greatly interconnected with a person's behavior as behavior is a higher intellectual ability that requires a person to have a healthy mind.

Stress is another factor that might be something very familiar to you. People think that stress can only affect the physical health of a person due to the rise of stress hormone levels and all the related metabolic changes. But, do you know that there are many changes occur in the chemistry of your brain, which might seriously interfere with the social interactions of a person? Yes, a stressed person finds it hard to build healthy social interactions as they are under so much of 'mental pressure' and once the stress is gone, the same person will find him building up good relationships with new people very easily.

A next important thing about social well-being is that there are special requirements it needs to fulfill in order to achieve the goal; A proper education, educating people about social interactions, fulfillment of basic needs, equality regardless of age, race, skin color or ethnicity and peace is some of the things which should be considered as essential to have a youth with a healthy social life.

IMPORTANCE OF SEXUAL HEALTH AT THIS AGE

Reproductive health, according to the World Health Organization (WHO) - is a state of physical, mental and social well-being for all items relating to the reproductive system at all stages of life.

Reproductive health is an essential part of general health concerns and personal aspects of life. Reproductive health implies that people can lead a satisfactory and safe sex life and that he is able to bear children, and is free to choose the conditions under which, where and how often to do so. But, in order to bear a child or have sex, an individual should be an adult.

The college students are adults as most of them are over the age of 16 and this is the time period in which many young adults start their sexual life. Saving the reproductive health of adolescents and young people is of great social importance. Reproductive health of today's children and adolescents who are in fertile age will directly affect the demographic processes in the next 10-15 years. The sexual and reproductive health of today's young adults will subsequently develop demographic situation which largely dependent on the concepts of family and marital relationships, sexual behavior and reproductive systems of modern teenagers after 10 years.

Reproductive health is closely related to sexual health, which, according to the WHO definition, is a state of physical, emotional, mental and social well-being related to sexuality. Sexual health requires a positive and respectful attitude to sexuality and sexual relationships and opportunities to lead a sex life that brings satisfaction, free of coercion, discrimination, and violence. Achieving and maintaining sexual health is inextricably linked to the respect, protection, and respect for the inherent rights of the people sexuality.

From a medical point of view of sexual life in physiologically, mature young men and women do not harm their health. The explicit physiological need for sex really has only accelerated in adolescents with psychosexual development. But, that does not mean a young adult is ready to have a child or ready to enter into a marital life. The eligibility of bearing a child and starting a marital life does not only depend on physical health but, also from mental and social health as well as economic state and living conditions of a person.

Even though sexual activities are considered to be activities of adulthood, in develop countries, many early teenagers becomes sexually active at a very low age such as 13 -15 years. Early sexual activity brings in a number of problems, one of which is teenage pregnancy. Anyhow, at the beginning of sexual activity, especially when it occurs at an early age (15-17 years), the risk of unintended pregnancy is quite high. Generally, this is because these individuals at these age groups are insufficiently informed on issues related to the unsafe sex and also because they do not always have access to condoms and other contraceptives.

Teenage pregnancy often ends in intended abortions. The frequency of complications after abortions and maternal mortality among adolescents is higher than in women older than 20 years. Immaturity and incomplete formation of an adolescent organism are a major cause of complications during pregnancy, labor abnormalities, maternal mortality and ill-health of children born to young mothers. That is why the young adults are not considered as able to bear a child even though they can get pregnant.

First of all, as young adults do not underestimate the importance of comprehensive preventive education on sexual and reproductive health, which will give them the knowledge and skills to make responsible decisions regarding their behavior, as well as building relationships, free from violence and based on mutual respect and gender equality. Numerous studies in various countries have shown convincingly that the fear that sex education can lead to a greater and earlier sexual activity among young people, is not justified.

Once again knowledge is gold; attend sex education campaigns and find answers for all those questions you might have. Getting to know about your sexual and reproductive health is important as you are stepping into the mature world. It is important that you get educated about having safe sex, contraceptive methods, sexually transmitted diseases and also the ways of maintaining sexual hygiene. But, the internet is definitely not the best place to learn all these things.

BAD DIETARY HABITS

Fast Food

Fast food is everywhere and everyone is walking towards this devastating trap. Each of us wants to make our life easy and the college students are not any exceptions for it. College students fall for this fast food very often and very easily. This is because; most of their time is consumed by studies, assignments, projects and so on. These are the different types of stresses faced by college students. What they do to distress themselves is just to feed themselves with tasty and spicy food. These tasty foods are fast food most of the time and that is because they are very tired to cook their own meals or have no mindset to cook or eat home food at all.

Even though some of the college students manage to do all sort of things like, sports, studies and extracurricular activities, most of them fail to balance their life. This leads to dependence on fast food as their main meals. Fast foods surely taste better than home food, but fast foods are loaded with extra sugar, fats, and bad cholesterols. What can this do to our health? If this habit of depending on the fast food continues for a longer duration, it may put the college life in a miserable situation where you might have to visit doctors at a very young age to manage your blood sugar, body weight and the blood pressure. This means regardless your age fast food can put your life in a risk.

A lot of energy drinks

A teenager without energy drinks are a rare thing. I can call it a fashion or a trend which is still surviving among college students. Most of them use this energy drinks to study whole night without sleeping or to do their assignments or projects throughout the night. Another group of college people is taking these energy drinks as a source of energy to play a sport.

These energy drinks are loaded with huge amount of sugar and caffeine. Caffeine and sugar are good when it is a small amount. However, energy drinks have 10 times more caffeine and sugar than it withstands by our body, which may definitely lead to disturbances of our metabolism. Metabolic changes put the person at risk for many metabolic diseases as if diabetes, hypercholesterolemia, and so on. In addition, insomnia or sleeplessness and hyperactiveness are the effects of excessive energy drinks consumption. These caffeinated drinks can cause serious effects on the quality of life.

Missing meals – Mostly the breakfast

Most of the college students think that the easy way to maintain their body weight or get in shape is through skipping a meal and most often, they tend to skip breakfast. Breakfast has become a choice and not a necessity. This is one of the worst mistakes you can ever do when it comes to meals. Let us see, what skipping breakfast can do to our body?

1. The stomach starts to digest itself. Regardless of whether or not we eat, the stomach produces hydrochloric acid, which is accumulated in large amounts from night to morning. What happens when there is no food to digest? The acidic secretions act on the mucosal layer or inner layer of the stomach and start to irritate it and the prolonged effect is mild gastritis to severe gastritis. This can be seen in people who are not already having gastritis but skipping breakfast alone. The stomach pain, heartburn, cramps in the stomach and other unpleasant sensations can be called as the first symptoms.

2. There is a stagnation of bile. The contraction of the gallbladder occurs only in response to the food that has got into the stomach. In this case, the gallbladder releases bile into the intestine, without which, the fats are not digested and not absorbed in the intestines. If the stomach is empty, the gall bladder does not work, bile "stagnant", thickened and forms into a stone. This leads to a painful condition known as bile stone disease. Generally, this condition needs the use of surgery to eliminate the stone from the system.

3. Do you know that skipping breakfast stops the work of intestines? The morning food serves as a boost or feast for the intestines so that the bile can help in the normal peristalsis. Peristalsis is the movement of intestines so that the content of the food can be moved from one location to the other. When this peristalsis cease, it leads to intestinal stagnation, abdominal distention (enlargement of the stomach with severe

gas, constipation and Dysbiosis (reduction of intestinal microflora).

4. Moreover, it is only with regard to the digestive system. However, the rejection of the breakfast, among other things, also leads to weight gain. It is proved that those who do not eat breakfast consume more calories during the day. After all, our hormones are also produced around the clock. The activity of metabolic processes is maximum in the morning hours. Usually, it is from 7 to 10 o'clock in the morning, regardless of whether a person feels awake or not. It takes place in the early morning with the release of the major human hormones: pituitary (prolactin, ACTH), adrenal (cortisol), thyroid (TSH) hormones that stimulate the metabolism throughout the body. For efficient operation of these systems the energy must be timely and optimally delivered, i.e. food. When there is no proper breakfast, all these systems stumbles.

5. If you regularly skip breakfast, the balance is disturbed in our body. The body will consume its own essential reserves for the body to run smoothly, and these stocks will not have time to recover. One consequence of this metabolic disorder is weight gain.

6. The activity of metabolic processes is high in the morning and in the evening is gradually reduced. If you skip breakfast, there is a risk shift in time and the remaining meals. We eat late at night when your metabolism in the minimal activity - get the deposition of nutrients as fat. All these events can put college students at heavy risk for gastritis, reflux diseases, bile stone disease,

constipation, gas accumulation, obesity, and diabetes mellitus and so on.

If you are not convinced, then let us see why do we need to eat breakfast?

- Breakfast is the main stimulator of metabolic processes, which gives the greatest amount of strength and energy to your body throughout the day.

- Proper breakfast helps to wake up, to focus and adjust the memory.

- Breakfast Regulates hunger and thus control weight.

- Healthy breakfast is inexpensive and delicious "medicine", which protects the body from diseases of the stomach, intestine, gall bladder, as well as obesity and diabetes.

- Breakfast improves mood and helps to cope with stressful situations, which in our life is immense.

HOW TO EAT RIGHT

Importance of a balanced diet

College life always redefines the definition of balanced diet. It is because most of them are not aware of the balanced diet and its meaning. Now you may think what does a balanced diet means? Let us have a look at the depth of the meaning of this word: A balanced diet is a diet, which provides the total daily needs of nutrients to our body in the correct amount; not less or not more. Balancing is the key to getting it right. A balanced diet should have it all, but, in the correct amounts and at the correct time.

We see many obese people and also many others who are weak and malnutritious. This is one of the best examples of the balance of feeding being broken down. Overeating increases the body weight and also the fat accumulation making a person obese. If you take one nutritional component more and the others less, it means, you break the balance of supplying nutrition to your body. Then what happens? There come the deficiencies. It might be calories or nutritional components.

The way of consuming food and the way of balancing the nutrition are simplified by the creation of the food pyramid. According to it cereals, grains, and starches that provide our body the energy, should be consumed the most, as we need a lot of energy to function. Then the fruits, vegetables, and greeneries should be the next. The third level of the food pyramid contains protein products such as fish, meat and poultry and also the dairy products and milk. The fats and the oils should be consumed the least.

Carbohydrates

The foods that contain starch are bread, rice, cereals and others. These foods supply our body energy and this energy is what keeps us active the whole day. Each and every second we spend the calories which we consumed from the food we eat. But, do not misunderstand these carbohydrates as refined starch. The carbohydrates explained here are non-refined starches and may include only about 10% of refined starch. Refined sugars and starches are the culprits of many metabolic disorders as well as cardiovascular diseases. The high heart attack, stroke, and obesity rate are mainly due to the consumption of many refined sugars and new researchers have proved it.

Next to carbohydrates, fruits and vegetables should be consumed the most. These fruits and vegetables supply us with enough of vitamins, minerals, micronutrients and a lot of fiber. These nutritional elements help our body function properly. Minerals and vitamins participate in metabolic chemical reactions which take place inside our cells, deactivate and eliminate all the free radicals which are byproducts of metabolic reactions, keep up our immunity and also protect our skin, nails, and hair. These elements are responsible for the beauty of our body outside as well as inside. The fibers in the vegetables and fruits help the bowels form proper stools and evacuate the remnants of digestion in a proper manner. There are also soluble fibers which optimizes the functions of the other internal organs such as heart and liver.

All the fruits are also packed with a whole lot of anti-oxidants and phytonutrients. These phytonutrients are micronutrients which cannot be classified as minerals or vitamins, yet, plays a major role in keeping our body healthy. The anti-oxidant content is very high in citrus than in any other fruit or vegetable. But, even the fruits contain a lot of antioxidants in the form of vitamin C, flavonoids, and anthocyanins. They help to remove the free radicals from our body. They fight against those components which can damage our cells and make us sick. And also, these antioxidants are good in stimulating our immunity and fighting against infections.

Anthocyanins are flavonoids found in some "blue-fruits" like blue-black grapes, mulberries, acai berry, chokeberry, blueberries, and blackberries. When making infused waters using these fruits, these anthocyanins dissolve and add a light color to the water. These pigments offer many health benefits. These compounds have potent anti-oxidant properties that help remove free radicals from the body, and thus offer protection against cancers, aging, infections, etc.

The next secret of fruits is that it gives us a glowing skin; A skin free of wrinkles, dryness, and pigmentations. Thanks to all those microelements in fruits. They are above any facial kits, creams, gels and to tonics. Once they go down the throat, they reach our skin; concentrates there, resulting a soft, smooth glowing skin.

Vegetables also contain a lot of soluble fibers than the fruits. They are very useful in preventing a rise in cholesterol level of the body and also if you are already in a diet plan, these waters may give a feeling of fullness to your stomach and delay your hunger.

Try adding three vegetables for each meal you consume and a fruit dessert to accompany the meal.

Proteins and fats

Next on the list is protein; meat, fish, eggs, dairy products, nuts, beans, and soy. Proteins are a necessary component of our body. It is needed for growth, cell regeneration and repairing of muscles and other organs. Keep in mind to supply your body with essential amino acids, when we talk about proteins. Essential amino acids are the proteins, which cannot be made by our body and is necessary to be consumed by food.

Meat is a very good source of proteins and Iron. The iron content in meat is presented as Heme (a form which is absorbed easily into our body). It is also one of the best sources of vitamin B12. Lean meat without skin is the best option if you are a meat lover. It cuts down fat and supplies you with a high amount of protein, iron, B12 and zinc.

Fish is another great source of protein and contains many minerals. The high content of Omega 3, 6 and 9 fatty acids is another reason to choose fish over meat. Omega 3, 6 and 9 reduces the cholesterol level and risk of cardiovascular diseases. It also helps maintain joint health and supply our body with a great amount of fat-soluble vitamins A, D, and E.

For vegetarians, the proteins of plant origin are the best. As vegetarians don't consume meat, fish or eggs there is a huge deficiency of protein and that should be supplied by proteins of plant origin such as soy, beans, and legumes. Even though you consume enough of plant proteins and fulfill the protein need, there is the risk of developing iron and B12 deficiency. Hence, it is best that you take supplements together with your daily meals.

The "Five a day" method is the latest approved method of eating. It says that you should eat five times a day. This five times consists of three meals and two snacks.

All the three meals should be balanced meals. The dieticians say that we should eat until we feel our stomach is 80% filled and not 100% or more. This will reduce many disorders of the digestive tract.

The time of the meals has an importance too. The breakfast, lunch, and snacks can be altered according to your wish but when it comes to dinner, you should be careful on how much you eat and at what time you eat. The Dinner is where the most people go wrong. The Dinner should be a light meal rich in vegetables and a few proteins. It should be consumed at least 2-3 hours prior to sleep. This prevents Gastro Esophageal Reflux Disease (GERD) and gastritis, which are the most common gastrointestinal disorders, which affects most of the college students.

Supplementation

Most of the college students do not concentrate on food, but they keep on studying or focusing on other activities and they fail to understand the fact that our body need nutrients to work properly. What is the possible solution to this problem? The solution can be the introduction of multivitamin supplements into everyday practice. The supplementary food plays a vital role in our life.

What do the supplements do to us? Supplementary food as if the multivitamins, helps our body to stay healthy. A healthy body has the power to perform its natural function more efficiently than your unhealthy body does. This supplementation of the multivitamins acts as the base to keep your body healthy.

Where can you get these supplements? It is possible to get the vitamin supplements from the food sources. If you cannot get these vitamins from your food, it is better to think about an alternative. This puts you in search of the best source of multivitamins available in the market with the help of your doctor. Moreover, you need to keep in mind that the vitamins should come from the natural sources. This is due to the fact that, our body recognizes the vitamins from natural sources at its best and readily uses them.

Habit of eating at home

Most of the college students face this problem of not able to cook their own food at home or manage it. The most important reason for it is a lack of time and college students seek something easy and give a huge energy flux to the body. This habit does not end up in good. The most important solution is to try to organize your time to prepare your own food at home. Home food is the best food because it does not contain huge loads of sugar or additives or taste boosters.

These special additives are highly dangerous and the major reason for obesity or overweight in college students.

Drinking enough water

Everybody knows that 2/3rd of the human body consists of water and that an adult should at least consume 2 liters of fluids per day. But it is also well known that many do not fit into this standard. But, we cannot forget that consuming enough amount of water is important for the life, health, beauty and slimming!

The water is the basic chemical ground for all human cells. It occupies most of the volume of each part of the body. For example, in the blood, there is about 90%, in the brain 85% and about 75% in the muscles and so on. Therefore, water is certainly the main medium for a human being's life.

When our body does not have enough amount of water, it makes an alarm by creating a condition called thirst. But, unfortunately, due to the fact that the majority of us consume only a third of the daily water need, most of us fail to completely hydrate ourselves and this leads to the development of many health conditions, which result by dehydration. If the body does not get enough fluids, it begins work in economy mode. First, it tries to provide hydration to the most important organs: kidneys, liver, heart, lungs, and brain by extracting water from the skin, intestine and joints, preventing any malfunctioning of these most important organs. But, what happens with the skin, gut and joints? Don't they suffer from dehydration?

Before making a decision of changing your unhealthy habits, it is always important to have a proper knowledge. Therefore, let us now have a look on what kind of role water plays in our body and what kind of role does it plays in maintaining or controlling the body weight. This is the most devastating problem of most of the college students.

The liver protects the body from the toxic effects of the food and medications we consume. Also, the liver is responsible for detoxifying the byproducts of microorganisms when we suffer from an infection. Liver's challenge is to deactivate the toxins and transform them into water- soluble substances, which, then will be eliminated from the body. If we keep proper water balance in our body, the functions of the liver become easy and thereby we get protected from toxic damage

The kidneys filter all kinds of body fluid. When a person drinks enough water, the kidneys eliminate excess fluid with the urine along with all the harmful substances. When a person consumes only a little amount of water, only a small amount of urine is formed as the body saves water for its main functions. Therefore, the urine becomes highly concentrated with the waste and when this happens for a long time, there comes the formation of stones in the kidneys and urinary tract.

Lymph collects dead cells and other waste, delivers them to the lymph nodes, where they are filtered and then sent for recycling in the liver and kidneys. And to cope with this responsible work lymph needs the help of normal water balance.

Moreover, during physical exercises, inadequate intake of water can be harmful to your body. When there is a lack of water, fatigue sets in quickly, coordination of movements gets disturbed, muscle spasms occur. Why does it happen? When a person moves actively, he sweats a lot and due to that, his blood volume decreases. If the liquid supply is not replenished, the heart finds is hard to pump the blood. Therefore, you should drink water before training, during workouts and after them, to avoid dehydration.

Among other things, water helps in shedding excessive weight and is also a key factor in losing weight. The water does not contain fat and cholesterol, it has no calories. Water reduces appetite and is involved in the processing of fat reserves. If the water in the body is insufficient, the kidneys cannot function normally. Then their role is handed over to the liver, and its ability to participate in the metabolism of fats is reduced. As a result, the fat begins to accumulate in the body and the person gets fat. Therefore, if a person wants to lose weight, but does not drink the right amount of water, the body will not properly metabolize fat.

You also need to recognize that often the body weight is increased due to water retention. For example, people think that if they drink less water, the body weight will be reduced, as the body will have a less amount of water. However, the result is reversed. If the body lacks water, it tries to keep every drop of liquid and puts it in reserve in the hands and feet. Therefore, it is recommended to give the body enough water. Moreover, you need to remember: The more salt people consume, the more your body retains water to dissolve the salt.

Insufficient water intake leads to dehydration. The dehydrated body cannot completely clean the harmful substances from the body and they are entered into the bloodstream. Thus, it is inevitably reflected in the skin. The skin becomes pale, flabby and scaly, with an earthy shade, pimples appear on the face, also, cellulitis appear on the thighs and buttocks and the heels and elbows dry out.

An average of about two liters of water is excreted by the kidneys each day, while the intestines, lungs, and skin eliminate fluid as well. If this amount of water is not regularly filled, then the body is dehydrated. To check if you are dehydrated or not, we can look at several signs and they are; fatigue, headache and muscle pain, dry mouth and dry eyes, intolerance to heat and dark urine.

The most frequently asked question is that how much of water a person should drink? Experts say that for the treatment of obesity, a healthy person should drink at least 8-10 glasses of water a day. In physical education or in hot climates people need to drink more water. An overweight person should add 1 glass of water for every 10 kg of excess weight. Keep in mind: when you are thirsty - it means that your body has already started dehydrating.

Is it possible to replace water with another substitute? Yes, of course. Drinking water can be really boring at times. Therefore, you can drink fresh fruit juices, vegetable juices as well as smoothies instead. Consuming tea, milk, and coffee has become a part of life. All of these things counted in hydrating yourself. But, drinking energy drinks, soft drinks, and alcoholic beverages will reduce the quality of hydration. They supply the body with a huge amount of calories and toxic substances, which can be a burden to our health. Try to enjoy hydrating yourself by adding new ideas and making it a part of your lifestyle.

IMPORTANCE OF SLEEP

Understanding Sleep

Humans spend more than a quarter of their life asleep. However, there are only a few, who actually know what sleep really is. Sleep is as important as food to a human body. The brain – the boss who controls our body and its functions regains its power when we are asleep. Many chemical reactions happen in our body even when we are still asleep. That is why we say that 'our brain never sleeps'. To live fully, to study and work, it is necessary to fully relax. In addition, it is also the object of special care provided and benefited by you. One of the main types of rest is sleep. It helps to restores energy reserves of the nervous system that are spent during wakefulness. During sleep, there is a coordination of physiological, biochemical and metabolic processes which connects the correlations between the functions of the various internal organ.

Humans have their own special sleep architecture, which can be characterized by 02 types of sleep;

1. REM (Rapid Eye Movement)
2. NREM (Non-rapid eye movement)

The NREM is then divided into 4 stages according to the depth. These cycles and stages of sleep are discovered with the use of electroencephalography (EEG) and have shown different EEG waves during different stages of sleep. Throughout the whole time of sleep, REM and NREM sleep alternate cyclically. However, it is not understood how these alternations function. The only thing we know is that irregular cycles and absence of sleep have indicated sleep disorders most of the time.

Normally the sleep begins with NREM stage 01 and then move towards stages 02, 03 and 04 in an orderly manner, showing that the sleep starts as falling asleep and continues to its depth. Then comes the REM sleep. Anyhow, a person never stays continuously in REM sleep, rather, cycles between stages of NREM and REM throughout the sleep. The greater part of the sleep consists of NREM sleep, while only 25% of the time is spent in REM sleep.

Sleep plays a vital role in a man's life. Getting enough of quality sleep will encourage your good health as well as help you function more. Moreover, sleep helps and supports the growth and development of young adults. The information that is being collected throughout the day is deposited during the sleep and there are millions of new neural pathways created in the brain in order to make new memories. Sleep also helps a person pay attention, make decisions and be creative. A lack of sleep can put your body in a huge stress as much as stress may disturb your sleep. Therefore, it is well understood that sleep deprivation can lead to many psychiatric disorders such as depression and suicide.

What is the quality of sleep?

The quality of the sleep encompasses the type and the characteristic of sleep. The quality of sleep cannot be defined clearly. The quality can somehow depend on the duration of sleep, the depth of sleep and the time taken to fall asleep. There is no limitation, which leads us to the exact definition of the quality of sleep. However, the doctors and scientist use this term to compare or to diagnose the situation. This method helps to determine whether or not you are suffering from sleeplessness and its severity.

REASONS FOR SLEEPLESSNESS

Sleeplessness or insomnia is a new age problem for most of the young adults, especially for those young students who go to college. Before asking the question on what to do? You need to understand the reasons for these sleepless nights and here are few reasons:

Circadian Rhythm

Every person has internal biorhythms of the day-night, called circadian rhythms. It stipulates that when we sleep, the quality and quantity of sleep changes according to your circadian rhythm. The more stable the circadian rhythm is, the more it can give you a better sleep. The cycle can be changed under the influence of various factors, including short naps, sleep, exercise, and exposure to light. Generally, it includes day-to-day activities from the dawn to the dusk.

Age

Age plays a vital role as a determinant in the pattern of sleep. The young individuals tend to be more active during the night due to the extra boost of hormones and due to their lifestyle. The scientific explanation is that the hormones definitely plays a vital role in causing insomnia and the extra energy which young individuals have secured in order to enjoy their nights engaging in many activities instead of rest. In addition, they do rest, but their pattern is completely different. The pattern of sleep changes every day and it is never the same another day. This is an important reason for the development of sleeplessness in younger individuals.

Psychological stressors

Psychological stressors such as tight deadlines, exams, relationship conflict, problems at college, can interfere with the sleep. It is very difficult to "turn off" all problems accumulated during the day. Everyone does not have the capability to turn off the daytime dilemma during night. Studying late night, remembering all of the events that have happened throughout the day, planning the next day (does it seem familiar to you?). In such situations, it is simply impossible to "turn off the switch" and plunge into fast and sound sleep.

Apart from studies, the major psychological stressor during college days is the problem with the relationship. The relationship does not simply mean an affair, but the relationship context is really large. The relationship dilemma during college years also includes the problem with your family, friends and definitely with your soul mate. Why do I mention soul mate? Everyone during their college years thinks that this is my soul mate. Some relationships were soul mate type of relationships, but most of them are not. The problem with the relationship begins from there. The misunderstanding can easily develop and this can be the major disaster during college years. Why do

I mention this? The statistics say most of the breakups happen during college years and the impact from it is really huge and it leaves a scar in a person. These problems can put a person to sleepless nights and even to depression. The depression is also a major reason for insomnia or sleeplessness. Therefore, this explains the high consumption of sleep inducing drugs during the college years. This is also shown by many statistics data released from many colleges.

Personal and social habits

Social or recreational drugs such as caffeine, nicotine and alcohol have great impact on the sleep hygiene more than it might seem at first glance. The coffee is the major supplier of caffeine. Caffeine, which remains in the body for 14 hours, the frequency of caffeine intake increases the wakefulness at night and accordingly reduces the amount of sleep. The sleeplessness induces by caffeine is presented at daytime with irritability and restlessness. Cigarettes and cigars are the major contributors of nicotine. The nicotine also possess the same effect as caffeine but the difference is that nicotine enters the body in smaller doses, begins to act as a sedative, and in large doses, they act as sleep inhibitor.

Alcohol can act as a sedative and it helps to fall asleep faster. However, since the processes of metabolism and cleansing of the body occur during sleep, it can make the person awake and do not give good sleep. The wakefulness can last up to 2-3 hours. Such awakening does not permit proper sleep. Moreover, the alcohol intake habit can cause nightmares, excessive sweating, and headache.

The other habits, which keep the sleep away, are watching TV late night, using computer or laptop continuously for more than 7 hours, engaged in emotional debate with your girlfriend or boyfriend and heavy eating before going to bed. All these can lead to the disturbance of sleep and in turn cause sleeplessness. The other common habits, which can affect the quality of sleep, are drinking plenty of fluids (beer or water) just before you go to bed. This can lead to the urge or the need to urinate when you are in a deep sleep. The frequency of this habit can disturb the quality of sleep and at last, it causes sleeplessness.

The other important habits of most of the college students are doing things at a wrong time. This can be greatly fit boys than girls. The boys at this younger age would love to build muscles by hitting a gym, but the college students are faced with the problem associated with time. Therefore, most of them choose to do heavy gym exercises at night. Generally, exercise can help you to fall asleep easily, but heavy workout as if weight lifting can put your body under immense stress and the pain associated with weight lifting and other heavy workouts disturb the sleep by increasing the wakefulness during sleep. This can cause poor sleep or sleeplessness.

NEGATIVE EFFECTS OF INSOMNIA

Any person at least once in his life faced with such a problem as sleep disturbance. The main symptoms of insomnia may be a lack of sleep, inability to sleep well, difficulty falling asleep, inability to return to sleep after waking up early. These unpleasant consequences of insomnia affect the quality of life; they have a negative impact on health.

1. Insomnia increases the risk of cancer diseases in future

   As per as the research, it was discovered that insomnia can lead to the development of breast cancer in women and prostate cancer in men.

2. Sleep disorder contributes to weight gain:

   The sleep disorder can affect the body by causing extra stress on the body and mind. Stress is very dangerous as this stress can lead to weight gain. The sleeplessness increases the stress hormone in our body, and this is, in turn, pave the way towards weight gain by triggering the hungry center in our brain. This sleeplessness leads to the development of eating disorder. Eating disorder can lead to weight gain by eating too much.

3. Development of anxiety disorder:

    This is the very much dangerous situation where if a person is suffering from another disease, anxiety disorder adds the chance of developing complications of that disease.

4. Sleepless cause depression:

    Another important effect of sleeplessness is depression. Depression can also lead to sleeplessness.

5. You become difficult to understand other people and control their emotions:

    Sleeplessness affects the relationship between friends or family members that have a negative impact on your study, relationship with people because you almost stop to understand other people's emotions.

6. The consequences of insomnia may be the development of diabetes:

    Sleeplessness contributes to the development of type 2 diabetes because it amplifies the body's resistance to insulin. Insulin is a hormone, which controls the level of glucose in the blood.

7. Unhealthy skin:

    If you cannot sleep, the body begins to produce large amounts of cortisol - a stress hormone. This leads to the fact that skin collagen deteriorates and loses smoothness and skin elasticity.

8. Insomnia reduces life expectancy:

    It is to prove that people who sleep a full sleep are much less likely to die within 10 years. A full sleep is considered to be more than 6 hours a day.

9. Lack of sleep increases the risk of cardiovascular disease:

    48% of the people who suffers from sleeplessness develop cardiovascular diseases as if stroke.

10. Insomnia increases blood pressure.

    Sleeplessness put the body through stress and as a result, the blood pressure rises. In addition, sleeplessness causes many problems associated with heart and it also can be the reason for increased blood pressure.

11. From lack of sleep weakens the body:

    It is because during a full sleep growth hormones are released that restores tissue in the body, help to increase muscle mass, bone thickening and strengthening the skin.

13. Development of chronic pain

    The sleeplessness focuses all type of pain in our body and this leads to constant pain throughout the day.

14. Memory loss:

    Memory is a delicate factor, which needs utmost care. However, sleeplessness put the brain and the total system at stress and this can lead to memory loss. This is highly problematic for college students as it is very much needed to recall what they studied in past year to have a clear understanding of advanced subjects.

PHYSICAL FITNESS AT TEENAGE

In teenagers, as in any others, physical activity is very important. The cardiovascular system of the body is subjected to show improved functions when you are physically active. Active physical exercises are especially needed for today's younger generation, who are forced to spend a lot of time in a sitting position - at college in the classroom and at home with homework. In addition, most modern college goers are addicted to the computer, mobile phone, and the Internet. These people do not want to do anything but to stay with computer or phone for hours in a sitting position. This is also due to the social Medias as if Facebook, Instagram, and Twitter and so on, which took over the control of these young adults to live in the internet age but to be away from physical activeness.

Physical activity

The young adults must be physically active for at least 60 minutes a day. This does not mean simply doing your day-to-day activities. Being physically active is defined as enrolling in a high-intensity exercise, which comes from a specific sports or exercise regimen.

In young adults as in college goers, the energy packed within them is extremely high and this is due to the efficient supply of energy from strong muscles. This strong muscles and strong body is the plus point of these young adults who are college goers. This enables these young individuals to make themselves more active by doing some kind of a sports. These sports or physical activity does not make you hit the gym. The gym is always not the endpoint of the word 'physical activity'.

These high active natural states give them the advantage of losing weight easily. This is clearly shown by the spontaneous growth of muscles at this stage. Think of a situation in which a person who is in his 30 and a person in 20, performing the same set of exercises. However, the result of the exercise on the body is greater on the 20-year-old person than on the 30-year-old person. This tells us the fact that extreme physical activity is not suitable without proper guidance. Therefore, this important factor should be taken into account when a coach or counselor when selecting exercises for a young adult. This shows us that the best set of exercises for college goers are short duration exercises or practising a sport.

How to choose a sport?

The most important job is to choose the correct sport for the correct person. There are various factors that has to be taken into consideration when choosing a sport. The first important factor that needs to consider is the physiological characteristic of an organism. This includes the appearance and the built level of a person. When you take a group of college- goers, you can divide them into various types according to how tall they are or how short they are. In addition, there are other factors as if how broad or lean they are and all these contribute to the selection criteria of sports. It is very much important to keep all these factors into consideration while making the choice of sport because the negligence of these factors can lead to fatal injuries. In addition, every sport requires guidance before beginning it. This is because wrong techniques also can lead to fatal injuries and can be life threatening sometimes.

Protein powders and health

Proteins are one of the important nutrition components. It is highly essential for the body. This is because proteins are the building blocks of our body. Proteins are highly needed in the growing period as it is needed in the development of our body. However, the proteins from the natural sources are the best source of proteins. Why these natural proteins are a better choice? This is because these natural proteins are easily digestible and converted into smaller units known as amino acids. Amino acids involve in many reactions in the body.

However, the gym is the advertisement platform for the artificial protein powders. Most of these protein powders claim that they are 100% natural. Nevertheless, these protein powders are packed with many chemical substances as if preservatives. All of these are synthetic materials and hence, they can increase the workload on liver. This is because the liver is the detoxification organ. Moreover, these protein substances are excreted in urine. Kidneys find it hard to filter it and thus these proteins disturb functions of kidneys.

This shows the importance of limiting the use of protein powders during any part of life. However, the college goers are very much famous for not drinking enough of fluids. The dehydration and protein powder intake together can put your kidneys at high risk of kidney dysfunction and in severe cases even cause kidney failure.

All these effects can be avoided by using natural proteins in your diet instead of the use of artificial proteins. The addition of animal products and plant-based proteins supply the body with the surplus amount of natural proteins.

What physical fitness does to our body?

Physical fitness does many things to our body. Enrolling in any sport comes with an added advantage of physical activeness. It is the very important benefit of physical fitness. The physical activeness is the refreshed and stress-free state of our body and mind. This is mainly done by increasing the secretion of the happy hormone - "serotonin" in our brain. In addition, sport or the exercise itself contributes to self-message the body and results in reduced level of stress. All these contribute to elevated mood, memory, and intelligence. It is highly required by anyone but specifically needed by college students.

In addition, the other features of the physical fitness are flexibility, stability, and strength. Total flexibility - this is the mobility of all joints, which allows you to perform a variety of movements with large amplitude. The flexibility also depends on the age. Usually, the mobility of large parts of the body is increased from 7 to 13-14 years and usually stabilized at 16-17 years, and then a steady downward trend. However, if after 13-14 years of age do not perform stretching exercises; the flexibility can begin to decline as early as in the adolescence age. On the contrary, experience shows that even in the age of 35-40 years, after regular physical exercises with the use of a variety of means and methods, increased flexibility, and some people reaches or exceeds the level of it, which was in their younger years. These are people who had a physical fitness or participation in sports or exercise during their teen years. This helps to retain the flexibility at any age. Moreover, the increased flexibility prevents injury, as if the body is equipped to bend ormove in the desired way.

In addition, the flexibility helps a person to achieve stability. Stability is also an important feature of physical fitness of a person and the person can withstand movements without causing huge changes. In addition, Flexibility and stability give a person with strength, which is an important achievement as a result of physical fitness.

THE STRESS

Are you feeling restless, tired or anxious? Are you feeling that 'it is too much' or that you 'can't handle it anymore?' If so don't worry. This is because you are simply stressed out. Stress is something whichthe student, have to go through most of the time during their college life.

Stress is not a bad thing. Students, of course, need a little bit of stress in order to show their maximum effort. We also can say that when people are a little bit stressed they gain their lost focus and concentration. Also stress can be defined as a burst of energy, which may make a person function at his best. Therefore, stress is good – but it is good only when it is there for a short time period.

The stress we hear about the most isnot the stress that break records, but, isthe chronic stress – the stress which continues for months and years. Yes, it is about the stress that we live with, in our day-to- day lives. This is the stress which we define as a very negative factor to maintain our good health. Chronic stress is not the stress that you find before an exam or a soccer match, it is the stress which a student carries every single day – It can be due to overwork, school problems, family problems and many others. This stress never has a positive influence on our brain or body. Itcan actually destroy our brain cells.

A chronic stress such as family problems at home or getting bullied at school may affect the functions of your brain. The causes of stress can be essentially anything that irritates him. For example to external reasons include concern for any reason (death of a relative, problems with friends). Internal stresses can be frequently getting ill and dependence for drugs or alcohol.

Stress and depression can be subject to both women and men almost equally. However, each body has its own characteristics. If you begin to notice signs that show stress in your body, it is necessary to identify their causes. It is quite clear that the causes of stress are much lighter than its consequences. After all, no wonder they say that "all diseases begin from the nerves."

When there is a stressful situation, the braincollects the information and collects these data in hypothalamus – a part of the brain that regulates many hormonal and neural activities. Hypothalamus then sends a signal to the pituitary gland of the brain. The nerves of the pituitary gland get stimulated as soon as they receive the signals from hypothalamus and thereby produce Corticotropin releasing hormone (CRH) which commands the adrenal glands to produce stress hormones. This seriesof information exchange between brain neuron cells and endocrine glands control the body during stress.

When the adrenal glands receive the signal to release stress hormones, the adrenal glands secrete a hormone, which is known as 'cortisol'. This is the hormone which is responsible for instant actions of a person when he receives a signal of acute stress.

Even though increased cortisol levels are good in an acute situation, a high level of cortisol in the blood for a long time period can damage the nerve cells in your brain. It is found that chronic stresses increase the activity and neural connections in the fear centre of our brain.

Cortisol, the stress hormone, can actually shrink your brain. When brain shrinks to an extensive grade, the nerves lose its synaptic connection, especially in the prefrontal cortex, which regulates behaviors such as concentration, decision making, judgement and social interactions. So, too much of stress can be a disturbance for good grades.

Chronic stress can result in depression. It is well known that depressed people have a high level of cortisol in blood. The neuroscientists now doubt that the chemical changes in the brain during depression are not a cause of depression, but a response of the brain to the chronic stress conditions.

When cortisol binds to the receptors of neurons, it allowsa large influx of calcium and excitation of nerves. It can even help a person cope with a life threatening situation. But, when this happen for a long time, the calcium keeps on accumulating in cells, making the nerves to fire very frequently. This lead to quick death of nerve cells, which literally can be called as 'fired to death'.

Now you must be thinking about how you can tackle this stressin the right way. Yes, I admit that it is not easy. But, is you can give a little time for ourselves and to maintain our good health, you sure can find a solution. But, unfortunately, many college students have a very busy lifestyle and do not find some time for relaxation. Anyhow, you can still do something about it. Have a weekend off, try one of these following methods of relaxing. I am sure that after a small break, you can bounce back with better health and better energy!

To learn how to cope with stressful situations, use a relaxation technique such as deep regular breathing. Give yourself enough time to recover from stress.Do regular exercises. Thus, you will improve your health and well-being and increase the body's ability to respond to stress. Do not drink alcohol or take any narcotics. Limit consumption of caffeine, because it can enhance the symptoms of anxiety. Learn how to confront their fears. Even if they did not work, meet a doctor for assistance.

MANAGING STRESS

College years are tiresome, stressful and troublesome. These eventsdirectly as well as indirectly induce stress. The overall effect of being highly active is the increased level of all types of stress. Most of us think that relaxation of a stressful day can be simply achieved by sitting in front of the TV or your computer and wasting time watching dramas, movies or playing video games on your play station. Actually, these habits only can increase the severity of the stress in the body. Our body tries hard to communicate with ourselves to say that these habits are masked as stress relievers, but they actually hide the stress for a short period of time. Our body is deteriorating as we try to hide the stress as the amount of stress is huge and the body needs to react to it. What can these college goers do?

There are various options available to relax yourself. They are collectively known as relaxation techniques. These techniques are deep breathing, meditation, rhythmic exercise, yoga, aromatherapy, reflex therapy and so on.

Adjusting the balance of your Nervous system

The stress reaction can be cruel towards your nervous system; as a result, your body secretes many chemical substances in order to prepare yourself for the sudden stress stimuli. This reaction is known as the fight or flight mechanism. These fight and flight mechanisms are natural response prepared by our body to survive in emergencies. However, the constant stress can bea turmoil for our health.

Avoiding stress completely is an unreasonable goal, but you need to learn methods to induce the relaxation response. These relaxation responses know the tricks to halt your stress response and to re- achieve the lost balance.

When you turn on your relaxation response, you may be able to find the following responses from your body:

- Even breathing and a more of a subtleinhalation and exhalation.

- The decline in the heart rates to the normal level.

- Relaxation of overall muscle groups.

- Decline in the level of your blood pressure and which sits within the range of normal level.

- Activation of self-healing of your body.

Moreover, these relaxation responses do not alone settles down the physical attributions of stress, but also increases the overall energy level of the body. In addition, the relaxation response also influences on the body's immune system and increases the body'sdefence mechanism which protects the body from diseases and disease-causing germs. That is not all of it, but also relaxation response helps you to have a keen focus with improved intelligence. College students always complaint that they are not feeling fit and with this relaxation responses, they have no more "not fit "option, but they are gifted with an elevated mood with an immense amount of self-motivation. These benefits can be harvested by anyone who performs the right set of relaxation techniques.

In the making of relaxation response:

Most of the relaxation techniques, which are used, have the power to re-balance the state of your nervous system. These relaxation techniques do not simply mean sleeping 24 hours a day and not doing any work, but these relaxation techniques are focused on penetrating into your body through your mind and the relaxation of the mind helps to coordinate the relaxation of the body.

The relaxation techniques are not difficult to learn, but you need to do your homework in order achieve perfection in it. The perfection of these techniques is very important, as the perfection is directly proportional to the degree of the relaxation response achieved. It is highly advisable to spend at least 10-20 min per day for your relaxation techniques. However, it is up to you to increase your amount of practice per day. Do not panic, most of the time, you do not need to sit separately and perform these relaxation techniques. These techniques can be performed when you are in your college or even during the breaks. It is your commitment that matters but not the location.

Which technique is for me?

You cannot call a single relaxation technique as the best technique. The selection of the relaxation technique depends on various factors. They are

- The need of a person

- Fitness level of a person

- The amount of stress

The ideal relaxation technique is the one which mingles with your lifestyle and with your body. In addition, ideal relaxation technique terminates the unnecessary thought generating process and leads to increased focus of the mind towards relaxation. Most of the evidence show that usage of varying techniques keep you enthusiastic and more focused than repeating the same technique and ending with boredom.

It is very important to know the way in which your body reacts to stress. This affects the choice ofthe relaxation technique, which is ideal for you:

If you are a person who expresses the stress with anger or agitation, the best way to relieve your stress is by calming relaxation techniques as if meditation, different breathing techniques, and progressive muscle relaxation.

If you are a person who is depressed or disconnected with stress, the best way to relieve your stress is by choosing relaxation techniques that can increase your energy and enthusiasm and they are massages, exercises with rhythmic movement or yoga.

There is another group of people who freeze at the very momentthey encounter with stress. These people need to transform this stage into anger or agitation state or as depression state. This helps in the further choice of the relaxation technique. However, the frozen state can be transformed by performing exercises that involve the use of limbs as if jogging, running, dancing and so on.

Incorporation of relaxation techniques into your life

The ideal way to begin and to follow a relaxation technique is to incorporate these techniques into your day-to-day life. It is certainly hard and challenging to fit these relaxation techniques midst of busy schedules, but most of these techniques can be practiced while performing other activities. For example, you may choose to perform meditation whiletravelling to college or while already in the college. You can use your breaks and naps to spend for this relaxation techniques and they are worth spending those times for.

Tips for incorporating relaxation techniques into your life

1. **Keep early morning for relaxation techniques of your choice in your schedule.**

   Early morning usually works for most of the people as the morning does not have any burden, distraction, or disturbances. This schedule helps to practice the relaxation technique of your choice regularly.

2. **Application of mindfulness when you exercise.**

Most of us try to watch or listen to music while we exercise. However, the more benefits you can add to your body by focusing on your body while youperform the exercises. Try to match your breathing with the exercise you perform.

3. **Do not practice these relaxation techniques when you feel sleepy.**

Most of these techniques are developed to relax the body in various ways. When you perform these techniques closer to your bedtime, it results in having a good sleep. These relaxation techniques are more effective when you do it a time where you are fully awake.

4. **It is alright to take a pause between the relaxation techniques.**

The pause can be for days or weeks, but you shouldn't be discouraged. You can start the relaxation technique again and can build the technique to a mastering level.

Yoga

Yoga is a type of relaxation technique, which is packed with poses as well as movements along with special breathing techniques. The Yoga is highly effective against chasing away anxiety and stress from our life and also yoga can improve your flexibility, balance, posture and so on. The continuous practice of yoga in day-to-day life also strengthens the output of the relaxation response that emits by it on the body.

What are the yoga poses or movements helps to chase away stress?

Generally, all of the yoga poses end with a relaxation pose. However, the best type of yogic exercises are one with slow poses which incorporate body movements, enables the deep level of breathing and stretching exercises are the best yogic exercises for stress relief.

- Power yoga – These are yogic exercises packed with intense poses and focus mostly on the fitness. In addition, power yoga is suitable for relaxation as well as for stimulation purposes.

- Satyananda – This is the oldest form of yoga and these are most suitable for beginners. This type of yoga is packed with mild poses, which are intended for deep relaxation.

- Hatha yoga – This is one of the mildest forms of yogic exercises and it is also more suitable for beginners.

Tai Chi

Have you got a chance to see a group of people performing slow and coordinated movements, then you have seen Tai Chi? Tai Chi is packed with flowing body movementswhich are slow and steady. These flawless body movements help to increase the concentration, relaxation and also help to circulate the essential amount of vital energy throughout the entire body. This form of relaxation technique is performed to calm the body and also in rechanneling the body which was disturbed by stress. It also uses the same principle of breathing as in the meditation and these breathing techniques help to bring the focus to one point.

Tai Chi is suitable for all sorts of people regardless of the fitness level. This technique similar to yoga, and can be practiced alone when you have learned the basics of Tai Chi.

Massage therapy

Massage therapy is not a new technique for relaxation purposes for you. Most of us had these massage at least once in the lifetime. In addition, these techniques do not need a spa or ayurvedic doctor. These techniques can be done at home or in your class breaks by simply adding some aromatic oil or essential oils, with deep breathing technique. These forms of massage therapy focus on spiritually massaging the mind as well as the physical body.

5 minutes quick massage

The massage therapy can be done by applying certain strokes on the group of muscles to relieve the tension. You can use your edge of your hands or with the help of fingers, tap on the place where the massage therapy is needed. You may also use the pressure points especially by applying the certain level of pressure with your finger on the muscles. In addition, you can also try to knead the muscles.

Begin the massage from the back part of your neck and also on the back part of shoulders. You may with your hand apply gentle pressure quickly all over the neck as well as on the shoulders. After giving the preliminary massage, you may use your thumbs to perform small circular movements on the base of the head or on the highest point of the neck.

The next step is to use your fingers on the scalp to tap mildly and this causes a huge amount of relaxation. The next step can be the application of the massage tothe face with the help of thumbs and fingertips by performing small and mild circular movements. Moreover, this short massage concludes by closing the eyes and applying hands on the eyes with proper inhaling and exhaling of air.

Meditation

This is one of the important forms of relaxation technique, which is performed by most of the people. Meditation is the proper controlling of mind, soul, and body through keen focus along with deep breathing. Meditation takes you on a journey similar to sleep, but the phases of the meditation and sleep are different. The meditation makes yourself reach deep relaxation by increasing the focus of mind, body, and soul. This type of relaxation technique is best suitable for college goers who have trouble concentrating or keeping their focus at one point.

A hot bath

A hot bath can do much magic including calming down the body. The hot water, which falls on our body, tends to remove the pain stimulus from the body. In addition, a hot bath increases the blood flow to the skin and hence, the circulatory disturbances of our body decreased. This helps the person to have an increased mood level or a good mood after a hot bath. In addition, the hot water massages the body from top to bottom and removes the tension of the muscles. Overall, a hot bath can decrease the physical and mental aspects of the stress on the body by giving a deep relaxation.

Aromatherapy

Do you know that smell can decrease your stress? Smells are perceived by our nose and analyzed in the brain. The translation of smells by our brain and of understanding it is a huge process. However, certain smells have the power to reduce stress from our body. This is especially true for essential oils. The aromas of these essential oils have a calming effect on the mind. Thishelps to achieve relaxation by calming the mind and helps the mind to focus on expelling the stress reaction from our body.

TEENAGE DEPRESSION

Suicidal behavior and depression can ruin the life of teenagers and young adults. In the USA, teenage suicide ranks first among the causes of death of young people and adolescents. Statistics show that every year 500,000 teens attempt suicide and 5,000 of them brought their attempts to death. These data are reminiscent of the epidemic.

Problems in the family, loss of a loved one, failure at school, or persistent failure in personal relationships, all of which can cause negative thoughts and lead to depression. But for a teenager, these problems seem insurmountable, and the pain they cause intolerable. Suicide is anact of desperation and has become the main outcome of teenage depression.

Teenage Depression - a "strange combination" you might say. Well, depression in teenagers and young adults are not rare and are there in varying degrees of severity. Unfortunately, the phenomenon is frequent enough, and at the same time insidious and dangerous. It is also difficult to recognize the people who suffer from it. And it is often detected too late when the tragedy has already occurred. The friends and family would say, the young man was always, almost the same. This is the danger and as well as the cunningness of teenage depression.

The reasons for depression in adolescents are enormous. Also, the consequences are very different, depending on the severity of the condition of a teenager - from failure and absenteeism in the school to suicide. That is why it is so important to know how to recognize impending trouble and to urgently seek expert opinions even if it regarding yourself or the other.

As an example, getting a bad grade can develop feelings of worthlessness and inferiority in a college student. School performance, social status among peers, sexual orientation, and family well-being are the factors that have a huge impact on the mental state of a teenager. Sometimes, teen depression may result from exposure to environmental factors. But if any friends or relatives- or even hobbies - cannot help a teenager get rid of feelings of unhappiness, regardless of its causes, there is a huge possibility that he is sick of teenage depression.

Often, teenage depression symptoms manifest as changes in mood and behavior. Sick children lose motivation in life and become withdrawn, they come home from school and just close themselves in a room and sit alone for hours. Such children have seen increased drowsiness, appetite swings and even criminal behavior, such as petty theft in stores or alcohol intoxication or drug intoxication.

Below are the main symptoms of adolescent depression:

- Lack of enthusiasm

- Persistent pain, such as headaches, stomach pain, back pain or a feeling of fatigue

- Inability to focus on something

- Difficulty in decision-making

- Irresponsible behavior - for example, forget about their duties, are late to school or skip it

- Loss of appetite or over-eating, which leads to significant weight loss or obesity

- Forgetfulness

- Obsession with thoughts of death

- rebellious behavior

- The feeling of sadness, anxiety or hopelessness

- Insomnia at night and increased drowsiness during the day

- The sudden decline in school performance

- The use of alcohol, drugs, and casual sexual relationships

- Avoiding friends

If this depression begins between the ages of 15 to 30 years, there is a high possibility that it can be hereditary. In addition, teenage depression is more common in those children in afamily where cases of depression were reported.

There are no specific medical tests, which help a person to say that the child is exactly ill with depression. That is why it is important that the depressed person is directed towards a psychiatrist in order to diagnose adolescent depression. Referring to the results of interviews and psychological tests with the teen, his family, teachers and friends, the doctor is able to confirm about the real condition of the person.

The extent of the disease and the risk of suicide, are determined on the basis of a detailed assessment of these interviews. According to the information obtained through interviews and psychological tests, the method of treatment is decided.

The psychiatrist will also consider the presence of other mental disorders, such as anxiety, schizophrenia or manic behavior. It also will examine in detail, whether the youth is capable of murder or suicide.

There are many treatments for depression, including the use of medications and psychotherapy.If depression is caused by problems in the family, an effective method of treatment can be a family therapy. Also, the teenager must feel the support of relatives, teachers and especially of friends to overcome the difficulties in learning and communicating with peers. In some cases, if the teen has a severe form of depression, there is a probability of hospitalization in a psychiatric hospital.

Depression might not interest you as you are in a good mental status, but, the people around you may not be the same. Remember, depression is always unnoticed and you may not recognize it unless you pay careful attention. I have seen how young adults regret when they find out their best friend has committed suicide just because he suffered from depression – and, above all, it was never noticed!

So let us see how you can help a person with depression, when you know he already suffers from it;

- **Be a good listener to them** – Communication is very important and listening plays a bigger role than speaking. The depressed person might have a lot of things to tell and nobody to listen. You can be that person who let him/her open up.

- **Talk at the correct time** – If you need to tell him something, chose a time when you both are relaxed so that the things you say will be more effective. Telling things when they are upset or when they fight can make his/her condition even worse.

- **Understand them** – Get more information about depression so that you can understand them better.

- **Encourage them to get help** – Encouraging them to get help may help them better than you help them by yourself. An expert can actually handle this condition and also carry out successful treatment so that your friends/relatives quality of life would be increased or back to normal.

ALCOHOL

According to research by David Nutt, a British psychiatrist, and pharmacologist, alcohol is the most harmful substance for humans. It is more harmful than heroin, cocaine, LSD, and other drugs. According to the statistics of the American Institute on Alcohol, 87% of people aged 18 and older had used alcohol in their lifetime. 71% consumed alcohol in the past year and 56% - during the last month.

About 20% of alcohol consumed is absorbed by the stomach. The remaining 80% go into the small intestine. The speed of alcohol absorption completely depends on its concentration in the drink. The higher it is, the faster the intoxication will be. A filled stomach slows down the absorption and the appearance of the intoxicating effect. After the alcohol has entered inthe stomach and small intestine, it is sent through the bloodstream throughout the body. More than 10% of alcohol is excreted by the kidneys and lungs through urine and breath. That is why alcohol testers allow you to determine whether you are drunk or not.

The rest of the alcohol is metabolized by the liver and so causes the greatest harm to the body. There are two main ways of liver damage when consuming alcohol;

1. Oxidative (oxidative) stress. As a result of chemical reactions that accompany alcohol metabolization in the liver, it may affect the liver cells. The body will try to heal itself, and because of this, an inflammation or scarring may begin.

2. Toxins in the intestinal bacteria. Alcohol can damage the intestine, due to which intestinalbacteria will be able to invade the liver and cause inflammation.

Alcohol effect does not occur immediately and it takes several stages. It occurs when the amount of alcohol entering exceeds the number that is excreted by the body.

Alcohol leads to fatty degeneration of the liver cells and impaired metabolization of vitamins, enzymes, protein and carbohydrates. Under the influence of alcohol, the properties and amount of gastric juice are changed, the pancreas is disrupted, which can lead to pancreatitisand diabetes. Even a light beer is a strong diuretic. And, if it is used regularly, the minerals and nutrients of the body might wash away, the loss of which for a growing teenager's organism may be irreparable. A sweet low-alcohol cocktail in jars is very popular among teenagers - a real explosive mixture of sugar, dye, and alcohol, which, in addition to a dose of alcohol, delivers the body of a teenager excessive amount of calories. Often in these jars contain caffeine that negatively affects the nervous and cardiovascular systems.

Blurred vision, slurred speech, body imbalance and memory loss is effects of alcohol on the brain. People often use alcohol and begin to experience problems with coordination, balance and common sense after about a year. One of the main symptoms is inhibited reactions, so the drivers are forbidden to manage transport in a drunken state. Alcohol changes the level of neurotransmitters, which transmit the impulses from neurons to muscle tissue. Neurotransmitters are responsible for the processing of external stimuli, emotions, and behavior. They can either excite the electrical activity in the brain or inhibit it. One of the major inhibitory neurotransmitters is gamma-aminobutyric acid and alcohol enhances its effect, thus making unstable and slow movements and slurred speech in drunken people.

Sexual intercourse without contraception among adolescents happen more in a "drunken" state. Such casual relationships can lead to infection with sexually transmitted infections, hepatitis B and C and HIV infection. Often, unprotected sex can cause early pregnancy among girls and abortion following him gynecological problems.

Alcohol violates the cardiovascular system by causing tachycardia and blood pressure drops. The immune system is no longer stable to carry out its functions and it is a reason for the teenagers catch infections all the time. Not only colds but, among young people who drinks, urinary tract infection and kidney failure and chronic inflammatory airway disease, is common most of the time.

At present, the many teenagers in the world celebrate the growth of consumption of alcoholic drinks. In this regard, in many countries more and more attention is paid to the problem of the spread of alcoholism among young people

French doctors have received even more alarming research results. Doctors have been studying the effects of alcohol on the development of the disease and found that there is a relationship between cancer and regular use of alcohol. They argue that if a glass of wine on adaily basis to take the risk of developing cancer of the throat or mouth increases by 168%.

How to reduce the negative effects of alcohol?

1. First of all the best solution is - stop drinking.

2. But, if you still cannot do it here are some tips to help reduce the effects of alcohol on the body:

- Drink plenty of water. Alcohol eliminates a lot of fluid from the body. Ideally, you should drink an extra liter of water, or even two, if you know you are going to drink alcohol.

- Eat. As already mentioned, a full stomach slows down the absorption of alcohol, giving the body time to gradually withdraw it.

- Do not lean on fatty foods. Yes, fats produce the film, which prevents the absorption of alcohol in the stomach, but an excessive amount of fatty foods would harm the body than it would save you from alcohol.

- Avoid carbonated beverages. Carbon dioxide contained therein, accelerates the absorption of alcohol.

- If you just want to support the company and do not want to get drunk, then the best option - one drink per hour. By following this rule, you will give your body time to ensure that alcohol is withdrawn.

SMOKING

The next bad habit of college students is smoking. Today, we are able to see many smokingstudents in front of a college despite all those awareness campaigns that are held to teach the negative effects of smoking. Tobacco products are prepared from the dried tobacco leaves, which contain proteins, carbohydrates, minerals, fiber, enzymes and other fatty acids.

Tobacco is a herb. Tobacco smoke contains more than 4,200 different substances, of which over 200 are dangerous to the human body. Among them are particularly harmful nicotine, tobacco tar, carbon monoxide (carbon monoxide), and others. Strong poisons, radioactive substances and heavy metals that can destroy human cells are also included in tobacco. Smokers accumulate these harmful substances in the bronchi, lungs, liver and kidneys. Products of dry distillation of tobacco contain tar andthis tar and chemicals are carcinogenic (benzpyrene). Smokers are 20 times more likely to develop malignant tumors of the lung, esophagus, stomach, larynx, mouth, and others. The longer a person smokes, the greater the chance of dying from this disease.

Up to a third of overall toxic substances, nicotine takes its own place.**Nicotine** is a drug that causes the addiction to smoke. Tobacco is one of the most dangerous plant poisons. The human lethal dose of nicotine is from 50 to 100 mg, and this dose enters the blood after smoking 20 - 25 cigarettes. A normal smoker smokes about 20 000 cigarettes for 30 years, consuming an average of 800 grams of nicotine, each piece of which is causing irreparable damage to health.

Nicotine enters the body, together with thetobacco smoke and is neutralized primarily in the liver, kidney, and lung, but waste products are excreted within 10- 15 hours after smoking. Nicotine refers to nerve poisons. In animal experiments and observations of smokers revealed that nicotine in small doses excites the nerve cells, contributes to more frequent breathing and heartbeat, breach of heart rate, nausea and vomiting. In large doses, it slows down and then paralyzes the activity of the central nervous system. Nicotine acts on the endocrine glands, causing a spasm of blood vessels, increased blood pressure and increased the frequency of heart contractions. The detrimental effect on the sex glands leads to the development of male infertility - impotence.

Carbon monoxide in the tobacco smoke causes oxygen starvation because it violates the ability of red blood cells (erythrocytes) to carry oxygen from the lungs to all organs and tissues. When smoking a regular flow of CO into the body, it leads to a decrease in respiratory capacity and limitationof physical activity. For this reason, the brain cells receive less oxygen, and thereby the mental capacity is reduced. It is clear that smoking is also incompatible with the physical activities and sports.

Tobacco tar is an extremely potent carcinogen. After smoking a cigarette it is clearly visible on the filter as a brown plaque. However, smoking a pack a day, even the so-called "light" cigarettes (in which the content of tobacco tar reduced), for the year a person puts into his body up to 700-800 grams of tobacco tar. It is not surprising that the lip cancer is 80 times common in smokers and lung cancer 67 times and gastric cancer 12 times more often than the non-smokers.

In humans, there is no organ or system, which would have no adverse effect of tobacco smoke and its other harmful substances. Smoker's central nervous system is in a constant state of tension because of the effects of exciting nicotine. But at the same time, it flows less blood (due to spasm of cerebral vessels), and the oxygen supply is dropped. Thereby, smoking reduces the mental capacity, weakens the memory and change the personality. In addition, the smokers feel an increased irritability and experience lethargy all the time.

Once in the airways, tobacco smoke adversely affects the entire respiratory system. Therefore, the harmful substances in tobacco smoke cause irritation of the mucous membranes of the mouth, nose, larynx, trachea and bronchi. As a result, it develops a chronic inflammation of the airways, often having colds, infections, and other disturbances of the tonsils. When a person smoke for 20 minutes, the action of the cilia and small airway mucosa is inhibited thereby it traps the harmful substances without being able to clear them. Prolonged smoking causes irritation of the vocal cords and narrowing of the glottis, which is why changing the tone and voice is often changed.

A typical sign of a smoker is coughing up dark mucus, especially in the morning. Also, smoking provokes the development of shortness of breath. Long-term chronic inflammation of the airways and lungs result in acute and chronic diseases, such as pneumonia, bronchial asthma, and bronchiectasis.

High blood pressure, disorders of cerebral circulation and heart attacks are common among smokers.

By stimulating the salivary glands, nicotine causes increased salivation. Smoker not only spits excessive saliva and swallow it but also send this nicotine to the digestive system exacerbating its harmful effects. There are other changes of the oral cavity such asthe destruction of tooth enamel, tooth decay, and the appearance of yellow plaque on the teeth, bleeding gums and loosening.

Gastric vessels are constricted during smoking, the gastric secretion is increased, and its composition is changed, appetite is reduced and digestion is inhibited. As a result of all these factors often lead to the development of gastric ulcers.

Only 25% of tobacco smoke enters the smoker's lungs, the remaining 75% are poisoning the air, causing harm to the others - this phenomenon is called "passive smoking". Hazardous to the health of non- smokers is to inhale the smoke of the other smokers. Passive smoking has 10 times more negative effects than active smoking.

Causes of addiction to smoking are different. At first, it is usually animitation, impress the people. Then in the process, a reflex of smoking is created and, finally, an addiction towards tobacco with dependence will be the end result.

The vast majority of smokers does not get the pleasure of smoking and is ready to quit this addiction, but refers only to the "lack of will". In fact, the main reason is a lack of motivation, purpose. That is why up to 99% of smokers, getting to doctors with serious consequences of smoking (myocardial infarction, stroke, brain cancer symptoms), immediately forget about smoking. It was found that more than 70% of smokers can quit smoking easily because they have no true dependence.

The fight against smoking and promotion of the dangers of smoking should start with primary school age, using all means (talks, lectures, movies, posters, etc.) to develop the student's negative attitude towards smoking. This work should widely involve parents, teachers and community organizations.

There are several ways to help you quit smoking. The most common of these is the use of nicotine replacement. This can be nicotine patches, gum, and inhalers. Their mechanism of action is the same, as they provide access to nicotine in the body But, they protecting the person from unpleasant withdrawal syndrome. Thus the effect of nicotine is retained, but the body no longer receives contained toxins in tobacco smoke. These methods can be used for a long time until the craving for cigarettes will be lost.

It is also possible to use special medicines for smoking (on doctor's advice). They do not contain nicotine and are antidepressants, restores emotional balance in the initial period of quitting. They can reduce palpitations and other negative symptoms associated with nicotine consumption.

Alternative methods of treatment of nicotine addiction include acupuncture (reflexology) and hypnosis. When acupuncture needles are introduced into the ear, they act on specific brain structures. As a result, the reflex of smoking collapses.

Very few people able to quit on the first try. If a former smoker lit up again, then the reasons are analyzed and the appropriate changes to the plan of quitting will be made in the next attempt.

As a teenager and a college student, you might have tried to stop smoking and even may have failed. But, it really doesn't matter. The change should start today and right now. If you feel you need support, your school counselor is the best person to talk to.Or even you can look up to your parents and relatives. Never give up on giving up on a badhabit as it can change your life. To enjoy a healthy youth, it is important that you follow a healthy lifestyle.

NARCOTICS AND THEIR EFFECTS ON HEALTH

It is believed that the term "narcotics" was first introduced by a Greek scientist named Galen and it used to describe the color of a substance that causes loss of sensation and paralysis. Anyhow, in medicine, narcotics are defined substances that have specific (stimulant, sedative, hallucinogenic, etc.) effects on the central nervous system.

Other than alcohol and smoking, narcotics have also become a concern in youth. There are many college students who are directed to rehabilitation centers to recover from drug dependence. That is why I thought talking about drugs is really important when it comes to college life.

Drugs have the ability to cause addiction and dependence. The dependence is manifested by withdrawal or "withdrawal syndrome, which is a hallmark of drugs. The withdrawal syndrome is associated with the termination of the regular intake of the drug and the accompanied restructuring of metabolism. The effects of narcotics can be very different: from mild discomfort or a burning sensation to the twisting joints, cramps, and severe pain.

People use drugs for many reasons; starting from a simple pleasure to live in a state of half- consciousness. Some say it helps to reduce their burden while the others say it's stylish to use drugs. Either way, these reasons are illusions and are myths. In fact, a person walking on the road who is addicted to drugs permanently exploits his best moral qualities. They change their personalities, lose friends, family and are unable to find a job and work or even study as he has lost his focus and concentration.

Narcotic drugs adversely affect all organs and systems, causing irreversible changes. Let us now see what drugs can do to your body?

Breathing is one of the basic conditions of life. During inhalation, thebody receives oxygen and during exhalation, it releases carbon dioxide. The depth and frequency of breathing are governed by the needs of the body. The regulatory mechanisms involve receptors that are excited by carbon dioxide. If the concentration of carbon dioxide increases, these receptors are excited, and nerve stimulation is transmitted to the respiratory center. Respiratory center increases the depth and frequency of breathing. This is what happens normally.

Drugs make the receptors insensitive, therefore when the accumulation of carbon dioxide occurs, the receptors are not excited. This, in turn, inhibits the excitability of the respiratory center. The addict will never be able to breathe completely. He condemns himself to a lifelong lack of oxygen (hypoxia). Addicts often die from respiratory failure through an accidental drug overdose. Death occurs within five minutes after the intravenous administration of the drug. Usually, help cannot be received on time as there are only a few minutes to save the life.

Choosing a narcotic is like choosing to strangle yourself slowly. The inhibited respiratory depression is really hard to store back.

A cough - a protective reaction that is useful in life-threatening conditions. A cough occurs when there are airway obstructions. But drugs desensitize the receptors, and thereby block the cough center in the brain. A man who starts to narcotics disables the mechanism of a protective cough. Additionally, he is also unable to remove dirt, mucus, and dust from his respiratory system and turn his lungs into a garbage bin which is packed with all these dirt.

Food is essential for life. Food supplies our body with energy and substances that are needed for growth and physical functions. Drugs inhibit the mechanisms of regulation of digestion. Drug users decrease all gustatory and olfactory sensations. They cannot fully enjoy the food. The appetite is reduced. Narcotics reduce the production of enzymes, bile, gastric and intestinal juices. Food is not fully absorbed and digested. Addict push himself to chronic starvation and therefore, typically, the drug addicts are underweight. Drugs cause spasm of the smooth muscles of the intestine and as a result passage of stool from one department to another is delayed. Then constipationsoccur very frequently. Decomposition and putrefaction process of food is being continued inside the gut itself and the produced toxins are absorbed into the bloodstream and spread throughout the body, damaging cells, causing their aging and death.

The mechanism of regulation of blood circulation is similar to the mechanisms of regulation of respiration. Blood pressure on the vessel walls are excited by receptors and desensitization of these receptors are responsible for reduced heart rate and circulation. For this reason, there is always a reduction of nutrition and oxygen which are necessary for the human cells and tissues. The functions of all cells weaken and after some time they are disabled. Thereby drug addict cannot work as usual as their body does not produce enough energy. Senile changes at a young age possibly visible.

For many mechanisms in addiction oppressed capabilities and needs. Gynecologists say that women addicts are marked with atrophic changes in the external and internal genital organs. Males also lose their fertility and come into a state of impotence.

According to statistics drug addicts are most likely to get infected with HIV and Hepatitis C by the means of needle sharing, blades sharing and by having unprotected sex.

Drug addiction is similar to a serious injury that could happen to you. The worst thing about it is that addicts realize their addiction too late and at that time they cannot live without it. Drug dependence sometimes develop after six months, a year, usually even in 2-3 months, but often a person becomes an addict after the first injection. The average length of a drug addicts' life is about 7-10 years. But there are many who die after 6-8 months after the start of regular admission.

Do you need these unpleasant changes during the best time of your life in which you would want to enjoy with friends and family? Do you still want to have an adventurous life in whichyou can experience new things? Do you have goals of reaching a higher place and be a successful person? Think twice if you are using narcotics or having an idea to use them. You probably don't want any drug to rewrite your life's stories. Say no to drugs and make your life a best one lived in earth!

HOW TO STUDY PRODUCTIVELY?

As college students, we live with the books most of the time. We go to school – we listen to lectures and when we come home – we study the whole night. Even though we keep ourselves so busy with the books all the time, at the end of the day, we find it hard sometimes to recall what we studied. Why does it happen? How can we study effectively? All these questions are unanswered. But, in this chapter, I want to write about those secrets, which the science believes to be the best ways of learning effectively.

According to Edgar Dale, there are many ways of learning and each way of learning holds its own effectiveness. After his researches, he developed a pyramid exhibiting the effectiveness of each method of learning named as "The Edgar Dale pyramid of learning".

According to him;

- Listening to lectures on or reading materials on the subject are the least effective ways of learning

- Teaching others and using experiences of real life situations are the most effective ways to learning

Now, let us have a look at some methods that increase the effectiveness of above-stated methods of study;

1. Writing notes

To make your notes valuable and more effective, you need to learn how to prepare them. As an example, when you highlight important events, dates and terms, use colored markers, it will greatly catch your eyes and will store strong memories in your brain. Use different colors as for the date - red, the terms - yellow and so on. In addition, learn how to summarize data using charts and tables, with objects associated with the terminology.

2. Compose summaries

Once you've written an outline, select the last page to write a generalized summary of what you studied. So it will be much easier to remember what you've recorded. Also do not forget to number the pages of abstract, ad number the reference pages in the summary.

3. Buy comfortable stationary

Comfortable pens, pencils, books and other stationary are very important. Organize them so that you can easily find them easily anytime. Buy small and low weight notepads and notebooks, so that you can carry them with you anywhere you can.

4. Take breaks

During the breaks, you need to switch to another kind of activity, for example, physical exercises or cooking. It is also possible during the holiday to listen to classical music. It is scientifically proven that the classics help us to concentrate on the tasks and motivates us to do things productively.

5. Attend additional courses

This will help you develop the necessary skills more quickly, and will contribute to your personal development as well. Make sure that the courses are following the same curriculum.

6. Reach the goal every day and not at once

It is proved that a small step a day eventually lead to big wins, so do not try to take it all at once, Carry your actions with positive emotions and visualize your achievements.

7. Grow in different directions

Do not concentrate on one thing, be a versatile person. This will make you an interesting person and a pleasant companion, and will contribute to the ability to find the right partners do your best. Attend workshops - learning new things are interesting. This will add pluses to your portfolio.

8. Do not be afraid to make mistakes

Life is designed in a way that you will be wrong at one time and correct at another. Therefore, adjust yourself to the fact that mistakes are experiences. In addition, remember that without a rain there is no rainbow! Therefore, do not pay much attention to your mistakes and failures, it is better to concentrate on and continue to move forward looking concentrating on your goal.

BRAIN BOOSTING

The pace of modern life, with its constantcongestion and stress, does not contribute to clarity of thoughts and mental performances. Inability to concentrate, loss of focus, lack of interest, weak memory are the clear signs of reduction of brain efficiency. How to increase the efficiency of the brain?

Increasing efficiency of the brain and its functions are well known by the term– "Brain boosting". This includes many ways that increase the brain's functions starting from its metabolism to its higher intellectual functions. Many students might have read different ways to increase their brain power and might have tried one or two ways to do so. But, I would like to highlight the fact that brain cannot reach its full efficiency only by a single method. The whole process depends on many practices suchas lifestyle modifications, brain training, practicing and much more. Let us have a look at basic rules of boosting your brain;

Make your brain sweat

Training your mind improves neural brain connection and creates a reserve of brain power. Do special exercises for the development of memory, begin to learn foreign languages, crossword puzzles and solve math problems, play games and educational activities.

Surrounded by all sorts of technology, we use our brain very rarely. Put the calculator and count in your mind, map your location in mind, without the help of the Navigator or try remembering phone numbers of your friends without looking at the notebook. These can be done easily every day. Start practicing today!

1. Eat right

It is known that the brain needs glucose to function well. Remember that it doesn't mean that the refined sugars are good as well. It is better to use products that contain natural starches such as potatoes, beans, rice, rye bread, nuts, etc. This food is digested more slowly and the brain has the energy charge for a few hours...

Next is Omega 3. Omega 3 increases your brain functions. Eat a lot of fish, eggs and nuts.

It is important not only what we eat, but also what we drink. Mug of coffee every hour- is not the best way to increase the efficiency of the brain. Put on your desktop with the usual bottle of water, and drink a glass every hour, even if not thirsty. This will save from heat and also from dehydration, which often lead to loss of performance and fatigue.

2. Do not overeat

The efficiency of the brain depends on the amount of food we eat. Scientists from the University of Florida, with the help of the experiments, have shown that satiety leads to dullness and negatively affects mental performance.

I'm sure many of you who overeat during lunch, feels like deteriorated afterward, and feels like sleeping. So, do not overeat!

3. Always read useful books

Reading not only increases the concentration but also stimulates the imagination: the contents of the book turns into our heads into visual images. Consequently, the brain works. "Any history book will let you make a comparison with the present that involves analytical abilities, under the responsibility of the right hemisphere "- says one of the researchers of the Mayo Clinic.

Instead of staring at the TV, grab some informative book and spend at least 30 minutes reading a book.

4. Relax and get enough sleep

Work without rest always leads to a loss of efficiency. Recently, American Journal of Epidemiology published a study of the magazine, which reads: "Fifty-five or more hours per week (eleven hours a day for five days) lead to a relatively low performance ontests of vocabulary and intelligence.

The main thing to do is to not to sit like a robot, and remember that if you are relaxed, it will increase your performance.

Do not forget to arrange a weekend and have a fun vacation- Camping! Hunting, fishing, hiking in the woods for berries, climbing mountains and barbecues in the country - all these are good ways to give your brain a rest from the stressful everyday life, recharge your batteries and increase the efficiency of the brain.

And, of course, speaking of the holiday and its impact on improving brain performance, it should be noted the importance of a healthy and proper sleep. It is known that lack of sleep leads to premature fatigue of the brain and lack of decision-making functions.

5. Give up on your bad habits

We have heard about the dangers of smoking and consumption of alcoholic beverages a lot, but there are people who claim that tobacco and alcohol (especially smoking), promote the efficiency of brain activity. However, doctors with numerous experiments proved that opinion about tobacco and alcohol as stimulants of brain activity is false and unfounded.

In fact, smoking tobacco and drinking alcohol does not only allow you to focus on your studies and work but also reduce the level of health, reduce the amount of work performed, as well as impair their quality.

Do you not know how to increase the efficiency of the brain? The first thing to do is to stop smoking and excessive alcohol consumption!

6.   Be active – move yourself

Daily exercise will help improve the elasticity of blood vessels and blood circulation, help restore lost neural connections and contribute to the emergence of new ones, which will lead to an improvement in brain efficiency.

7.   Do a head massage

Head and neck massage improves blood flow in the cerebral cortex and therefore useful for cell cerebral circulation. You can find information about how to do a self-massage of the head and neck area on the Internet if you couldn't ask a professional. If you do a head and neck massage daily for ten minutes for a few weeks, you will notice that your ability to think clearly will be improved and that your lost focus is regained.

8.   Use color and aromatherapy

It is proved that some of the smells and the colors have a calming effect, while others, on the contrary, are the stimuli to the brain. According to researchers, the brain stimulates good by the yellow color - it tones and invigorates, improves mental performance (you can hang above the desk drawing, in which the predominant color).

Aromatherapy uses your olfactory nerves to stimulate or relax the brain. There are certain odors that increase the efficiency of the brain and they mostly smell with woody citrus flavors. Use natural essential oils instead of air fresheners, as they function well as substances of aromatherapy. You can simply hand a packet of flower petals in your room, light an aroma candle or use soaps and toiletries with real essential oils. Try and see the difference!

GETTING RID OF YOUR ACNE

Teenage acne is the most widely discussed among all kinds of acne in different age groups. After all, it starts as a fearful side effect of growing up. There are many teenagers and young adults who have been frustrated with this condition as it affects their appearance as well as their self-confidence. Therefore, Acne is always not taken so light, when it comes to the teenagers. In the recent times, the dermatologists have described it as a disease that needs medicine, proper hygiene as well as mental support.

Now let us see what causes this nastyAcne:

1. During the period of puberty and adolescence, there is a surge of sexual hormones. It is believed that this disbalance of hormones, especially of testosterone and estrogen is the main cause of acne in young girls and boys.

2. The next is that, at this age, even your sebaceous glands function excessively making your skin oily. Then the sebum clogging of the pores take place and result in pimples.

3. The doctors also believe that acne can also result in bacterial infection, hence should be treated as an infection.

4. Hot sun, excessive sweating, dusts and low level of hygiene can be indirect causes of acne.

5. Stress above all can also result in aggressive spread of pimples. People who have uncontrolled stress get pimples in their face, neck and even in the shoulders.

As you know the symptoms, now let us see the main mistakes you do when you get acne;

1. Many people think acne in young people is something to ignore and not to worry about. This is actually the first mistake you do. If you can get treated for acne inits early phases, the complications would be reduced.

2. Do not press pimples. That's one of the main mistakes we do. Squeezing these pimples can make your acne worse. The bacteria in it can spread and also it will leave a scar. If you want to burst a pimple and clean it up, do it in the right way.

3. The next is to forget about your skin hygiene. Even though you have pimples, you might be simply using your old face wash, oily face cream and so on. This is a great risk of increasing the already existing pimples. Be careful of what you use and how clean your skin is if you have even one pimple.

Getting rid of teenage acne is not easy, but by keeping a set of rules, it can be done easily. The key to this treatment is to bring the situation under control so that the new spots will not appear.

To the best remedy for teenage acne include:

1. Salicylic acid. Perhaps the most popular tool, but also very effective if used correctly. This is included in most of the anti-acne face washes and gels.

2. Tar soap. Also very, very effective and it may effectively reduce your acne if you use it daily.

3. Try to keep to a low-fat diet and give up certain foods. Normalization of digestion will reduce the appearance of new spots on your skin. High sugar and oily food causes acne and so do the chocolate, coffee, and soft drinks. Staying away from them will keep you out of acne.

4. Wash your face at least two times a day with a cleanser or an anti-acne face wash. Cleaning the dirt and oil from your skin will reduce the inflammatory process as wellas the bacteria.

5. Vitamin D. Exposing 10 minutes to morning sun will provide you with enough of vitamin D. According to researchers, lack of vitamin D can also lead to acne.

6. Hot steam you face once in every 2 weeks and cleanse with lukewarm water afterwards. This helps the clogged pores to open up and self-clean all the dirt within. But,

do not hard scrubs if you have a pimple as it will cause scars. Once you steam, you can remove the pus out of your pimple using an extractor.

7. Just do not over think. It is believed that stress increases this condition and that is why people say their pimples increases when they study for an exam or when they have some personal problems. We know that our brain controls our total body and especially the hormone levels. As I have mentioned above, disbalance of hormones can cause pimples.

8. If nothing works out, then you have the best option of going to a dermatologist who will help you get rid of it. He will use vitamin A creams, antibiotics, and even some other medications to treat this so called acne, medically.

Acne surely is a common condition in youth, but it is never a condition to be left out without any treatment. The treatment depends on the severity, length, and cause of acne and anyhow requires you to maintain a proper hygiene of the skin.

Here are some tips to maintain proper skin hygiene;

1. Wash your skin at least two times a day; Morning after getting up and when you come home after being out.

2. Use a face cream that matches your skin type. For oily skin– non-oily creams, for dry skin – moisturizes and for sensitive skin - a cream for sensitive skin.

3. Use a face wash or soap that will cleanse your skin. Cleansers pull out the dirt in the pores of your skin.

4. Scrub your skin at least one time a week, so that all the deadcells will be removed.

5. As I have mentioned above hot steaming of skin can be helpful too.

6. Give a light massage whenever you can, it will increase the blood circulation of the skin. Thereby, you will get a healthy and a glowing skin.

7. Do not use all kinds of cosmetics you get in your hand. Before using a cosmetic, see how your skin reacts to it. Some people get allergies while some get pimples. Always be careful with your skin when it comes to cosmetics.

8. Treat your dandruff, as dandruff, can be another causeof acne that will frustrate you.

Hope you have enough tips to get rid of your acne now!

BEING SEXUALLY HEALTHY

High sexual activeness at this stage

What does it mean, "Being sexually healthy"? It is a vast topic, and this can be explained by the fact that these college goers are maintaining highly active sex life. College years are those years marked with full sexual maturation in every way including physical and mental attributes of the sex organs. This age makes everyone to push their limits and to experiment with varieties. The primary reason for this type of behavior is the hormonal changes. The college goers are boosted with the high amount of sex hormones in their body. These hormones do not leave anyone alone but speak within everyone to fantasize or to involve with the sex life. It is not abnormal to feel the urge to have sex, but how do you do it, which is the major question.

Sex life is not just about having sex whenever you want, but it is about a physical and emotional connection you make with a person. However, the hard part of the sex life is most of the college goers are not interested in making such connection. You may initially assume that it is not a problem, but the feelings, which you suppress when you avoid such connection, will be a troublesome remnant for your future. But, most of the college goers seem to change partners, and they advance in the amount and the way they get pleasure. Sex became a pleasure- inducing act regardless of whom you have sex. This extreme behavior is very common among college goers due to lack of knowledge and little awareness about the consequences they will be facing in the future.

This detached sexual act can harm the way they think and cause further problems with conflict within ourselves. But, the college students are interested in trying all types of sex, and even they go to extremes. This is not a healthy behavior. This can cause serious health problems as well. It is only few who can maintain a balance between their sex life and their love life. These are not philosophies but are essential facts which college goers should be brought into notice to avoid the unhealthy sexual behavior.

Understanding your sexual attractions

Before you understand sexual attractions, you need to know, what sexual attraction is and what causes it. Sexual attraction is something you connect defines, but you can feel it. This gives us a conclusion that the sexual attraction, which we experience mostly, is a physical attraction or shallow attraction. This means when you see beautiful women with the incredibly attractive body; your eyes at least once would glare at that women. This is a physical part of sexual attraction. The emotional part of the sexual attraction or deep attraction is something stronger, and it takes the time to develop. The emotional part of the sexual attraction is the personality and the intellectuality of the person. This type of attraction is highly essential to have a long- term relationship. This helps to understand your sexual attraction, and this answers many questions, which arises within you.

Risk of having multiple sexual partners

Sex life is fun, and a person who does not have much knowledge about sex life tends to overdo sex. What they do is change partners. At the end of the day, they had multiple sexual partners. Multiple sexual partners are not good news. Because a person with multiple sexual partners are at a greater risk for the development of sexually transmitted diseases. These are a special type of infections and are highly dangerous to us. When you have multiple partners, this disease circulates with your entire partners and at the end, all of your partners ended up having STDs or sexually transmitted diseases.

Sexually transmitted diseases are not a joke. They are highly aggressive in nature and most of the STDs cannot be cured but can only be controlled or prevented. Also, these STDs can cause serious effects if it is not diagnosed earlier. The long-term consequence of the STDs can be life threatening.

Moreover, another disease, which shakes the world, is AIDS. Multiple partners increase the chance of getting HIV infection. Everyone knows that the AIDS cannot be treated, but it can be controlled for a shorter duration.

How can you avoid all these infections? The first step is to avoid multiple partners. There are other ways in which these infections can be prevented by using proper contraceptive methods.

CONTRACEPTION

Contraception or contraceptive measures consist of a greater variety of choices. Each of these below-mentioned methods has their advantages, and they are

1.   Birth controlling pills

     There are two types of birth controlling pills such as combined oralcontraceptive pills and Progestin-only pills. Combined oral contraceptive pills have two hormones (estrogen and progestin), while Progestin-only pills contain progestin alone. They stop ovulation and inhibition of sperms movement as well as they make the cervical mucus thicker so that the sperms cannot get in. About 8% can get an accidental pregnancy in their first year.

     Tablets with combination oral contraceptives should be taken once a day for three weeks. The dormant (inactive) tablets may also be included in the packaging for the reception during the week when the combined pill is not taken to establish the habit of receiving one pill every day. The progestin-only pill must be taken every day of the month. However, skipping of the tablets can result in pregnancy. The tablets containing only progestin frequently cause irregular bleeding, so they are usually prescribed only in those cases where estrogen can be harmful.

The use of oral contraceptives also reduces the frequency of menstrual pain, premenstrual syndrome, irregular bleeding (in women with irregular menstrual periods), anemia, cysts, breast, and ovarian, tubal pregnancy (varieties of ectopic pregnancy), and inflammation of the fallopian tubes. In women taking oral contraceptives, there is also a less chance of rheumatoid arthritis and osteoporosis in the future.

2. Condoms

Nowadays condoms are considered the safest and most reliable means of contraception, which, unlike pharmacological preparations, does not cause side effects. Condoms are available to everyone: you can buy in any supermarket or drugstore. The cost of condoms is low. Of course, there are luxury condoms, but most of it is oriented to buyers with average incomes, which does not affect the quality of the goods.

However, when buying condoms you must always take into account some of the nuances:

- **Size -** As a rule, it's interesting to consumers in the first place, but often this information is not available, or it is false.

- **Thickness -** It affects the feeling, but practice shows that this concept is entirely subjective. Although, in some cases, this parameter is important for women:

in ultra- thin condoms, a person can feel better the warmth of the head of the penis;

- **The special shape** - These condoms are divided into several categories: ribbed, with edges in the form of rings, with pimples. Meets and combined version in which the ribs in the head combined with pimples at the base. Also, there are condoms with ribs located along (from the head to the base).

- **Lubrication** - At present, not lubricated condoms cannot be found anywhere. However, in any case before the condom buying better check availability on the package label "Lubricated". Additional protection against unwanted pregnancy and sexually transmitted infection in the event of rupture of condoms can provide by the lubricant that contains spermicide.

- **Reliability** - Condom use is accompanied by two main problems, slippage or rupture. The rupture of the condom is a serious issue. However, the lubrication with spermicide can prevent pregnancy. Also, the reasons behind rupture are low-quality lubrication and very frequent moves, so the severe friction results in the rupture. The slippage of the condom also depends on the lubrication.

- **Shelf life** - Typically, the shelf life of condoms is five years. Some condoms are suitable for use only for three years. Most often, condoms are sold after 12-15 months from the time of manufacture.

3.   Cervical cap

A small cap made from latex. It is applied with spermicides and inserted into the vagina and then the cervix so that the sperms would not enter the womb. About 16% can get an accidental pregnancy in their first year. Condoms

It is made from Latex or Polyurethane. Prevent pregnancy as well as STD (Sexually Transmitted Diseases) as it prevents body fluids from mixing. Condoms are worn by men before a sexual contact.

4.   Contraceptive Films

It is 2" X 2" sized thin film made with a spermicide and should be placed near the cervix. It is dissolved within seconds, and about 29% of women can get an accidental pregnancy in their first year.

5.   Contraceptive foam

This is placed in the vagina using an applicator. It kills sperms and blocks semen from entering cervical canal. About 29% of women can get an accidental pregnancy in their first year. Contraceptive foam is most useful when it is used together with a condom.

6.   Contraceptive implants

A single implant inserted into the upper arm. It gives away a hormone much likely progesterone. 5 out of 1000 women face an accidental pregnancy in their first year.

7. Contraceptive sponge

    It is a vaginal sponge and prevents semen from entering the cervix. Contraceptive sponges are highly effective in women when they have never given birth. About 16% of women can get an accidental pregnancy in their first year.

8. Diaphragm

    A diaphragm is a latex disc placed into a vagina. It should be left in the vagina for about 6-24 hours after the intercourse. The spermicide in diaphragm kills sperms. But, about 16% of women can get an accidental pregnancy in their first year.

9. Emergency contraception

    Emergency contraception is also known as the morning-after pill or Plan B. It can prevent pregnancy up to 5 days after unprotected sex. It is a stronger dose of the same hormones in birth controlling pills. Emergency contraception works best if you take it within 24 hours of sex.

10. Female condom

    It is a condom worn by women and has a 21% ratio of getting an accidental pregnancy in their first year.

11. Injectable contraceptives (Depo - Provera)

    This injection is administered every three months, and it helps toprevent ovulation while it has a 3% of failure rate.

Even though this method is only prescribed in severe cases, but most of the college goers prefer this method as the fact that this injection needed to take once in 3 months, so that the chance of missing Oral pills are avoided with the usage of this Depo injections.

12. Intrauterine contraception

Intrauterine emergency contraception is the intrauterine device (IUD) in the first 5-7 days after unprotected intercourse to prevent implantation of a fertilized egg already.

The method is slightly more efficient than the method of hormonal emergency contraception, but in its application should take into account the individual characteristics of the woman, her desire to continue for a long time to use this method of protection from unwanted pregnancy, as well as all possible contraindications to the introduction of an intrauterine device.

Ineffective birth controlling

Another problem of the college goers are that the amount of knowledge they have about birth controlling methods are very low. Due to that, they use these contraceptives in a way that these contraceptives will not function as a birth controlling method. This is the reason for increased number of pregnancy cases among college goers. What are the fates of such pregnancy? Most of the pregnancies end up in abortion.

Abortion can be a timely solution, but the future effect of abortion is highly negative. This is because; abortion leaves the person with many diseases for the future. This also predisposes the person to develop even cancer. In the meantime, abortion can also be highly dangerous to the mother.

Therefore, the birth controlling methods can prevent any unwanted pregnancies and abortions that can cause harm. Also, learning about this is not something to be shy about or something to hide out. A good sexual health is a part of your overall health and is a sole responsibility of you to keep it in a good state. Also don't forget that only male condoms can keep you out of sexually transmitted diseasesand unwanted pregnancies at the same time, even though all the other methods can keep you out of an unwanted pregnancy.